nice!

# Nacho Average

hello

Bye

belongs to: ______

Made in the USA
Monee, IL
18 October 2022

16135859R00061